AF528231

The Essential Guide to Cardiovascular Health

Sarvajna Akkineni

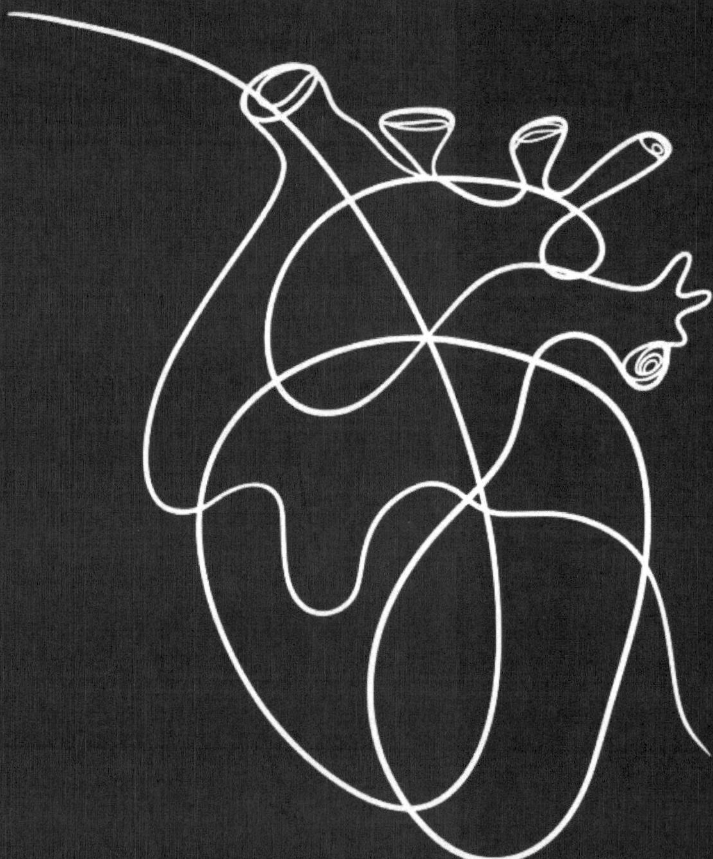

The Essential Guide to Cardiovascular Health

Sarvajna Akkineni

walnutpublication.com

INDIA • UK • USA

Copyright © Sarvajna Akkineni, 2025

All rights reserved. No part of this publication may be reproduced, stored in a retrieval system, or transmitted in any form or by any means, electronic, mechanical, recording or otherwise, without the prior written permission of the author.

This book has been published with all reasonable efforts taken to make the material error-free after the consent of the author. The author of this book is solely responsible and liable for its content including but not limited to the views, representations, descriptions, statements, information, opinions and references ["Content"]. The publisher does not endorse or approve the Content of this book or guarantee the reliability, accuracy or completeness of the Content published herein. The publisher and the author make no representations or warranties of any kind with respect to this book or its contents. The author and the publisher disclaim all such representations and warranties, including for example warranties of merchantability and educational or medical advice for a particular purpose. In addition, the author and the publisher do not represent or warrant that the information accessible via this book is accurate, complete or current.

Paperback ISBN: 978-93-48945-25-9
eBook ISBN: 978-93-48945-51-8

First Published in October 2025

Published by Walnut Publication

(an imprint of Vyusta Platforms Private Limited)

www.walnutpublication.com

India

Unit# 909, 9th Floor, Wave Silver Tower, Sector-18, Noida - 201301

UK

71-75 Shelton Street, Covent Garden, London, WC2H 9JQ, UK

Distributed by

ZopioTail

Disclaimer

The information provided in this book is intended for general informational and educational purposes only and is not a substitute for professional medical advice, diagnosis, or treatment. The content is designed to support, not replace, the relationship that exists between a patient and their physician or other qualified healthcare provider.

Always seek the advice of your physician or another qualified health professional with any questions you may have regarding a medical condition. Never disregard professional medical advice or delay in seeking it because of something you have read in this book. If you think you may have a medical emergency, call your doctor or emergency services immediately.

The author, editor and publisher have made every effort to ensure that the information contained herein is accurate and up-to-date at the time of publication. However, medical knowledge is constantly evolving and this book should not be considered a complete source of information on any topic. The author and publisher disclaim any liability for any direct or indirect loss or damage that may be suffered by any person as a result of the use or misuse of the information contained in this book. Reliance on any information provided in this book is solely at your own risk.

Preface

Cardiovascular diseases are the leading cause of death globally and their impact in India is profound and growing. Every day, countless individuals and families are affected by conditions like heart attacks, strokes and high blood pressure. Yet, for many, the world of heart health can feel complex and overwhelming, filled with medical jargon and confusing information.

This book was written to change that. My goal is to provide a clear, comprehensive and accessible guide to understanding the heart and the diseases that affect it. I believe that knowledge is power and by empowering patients, caregivers and the general public with reliable information, I can help people take control of their health, make informed decisions and work more effectively with their healthcare providers.

From the basics of how the heart works to detailed explanations of common conditions, diagnostic tests and treatments, this book is designed to be your trusted companion on your journey to better heart health. It is a resource born from the desire to demystify cardiovascular disease and to offer hope and clarity to all those who seek it.

Author
Sarvajna Akkineni

Introduction

The heart is the engine of the body, a remarkable muscle that works tirelessly every second of every day to pump life-sustaining blood to every organ and cell. When this vital organ is affected by disease, the consequences can be far-reaching and serious. "Cardiovascular diseases" is a broad term for a group of conditions that affect the heart and blood vessels, including:

- **Ischemic Heart Disease:** Caused by narrowed heart arteries.
- **Hypertensive Heart Disease:** Heart problems caused by high blood pressure.
- **Arrhythmia:** Irregular heartbeats.
- **Stroke:** A "brain attack" caused by a disruption of blood flow to the brain.
- **Rheumatic Heart Disease:** Damage to the heart valves from a previous infection.

Understanding these conditions—their causes, symptoms and risk factors—is the first step toward prevention and effective management. In recent decades, medical science has made incredible strides in diagnosing and treating heart disease, making it possible for many people to live long, healthy lives, even after a diagnosis.

This book will walk you through each of these major cardiovascular conditions in a clear and straightforward way. We will explore how these diseases develop, what you can do to prevent them and how to recognize the warning signs that require immediate attention. We will also demystify the medical tests and treatments you may encounter, so you can feel confident and prepared at every stage of your healthcare journey.

How to Use This Book

This guide is designed to be a flexible and user-friendly resource for readers of all backgrounds. You do not need a medical degree to understand the information inside. Here are a few tips on how to get the most out of this book:

- **Read it Your Way:** You can read the book from start to finish to get a complete overview of cardiovascular health, or you can jump directly to the chapters that are most relevant to you or your loved ones.
- **Consistent Chapter Structure:** Each chapter on a specific disease follows the same easy-to-navigate format: an introduction to the condition, followed by sections on symptoms, risk factors, diagnosis, treatment and prevention. This structure makes it easy to find the information you need quickly.
- **Quick Points:** At the end of each chapter, you will find a "Quick Points" summary that highlights the most essential takeaways.
- **Glossary of Terms:** If you come across a medical term you don't understand, you can refer to the comprehensive glossary at the end of the book for a simple, clear definition.
- **A Tool for Conversation:** We encourage you to use this book as a resource to prepare for appointments and to have more informed, productive conversations with your doctor.

Write down your questions and take this book with you to your next visit.

Our hope is that this guide will serve not just as a source of information, but as a source of confidence and empowerment for you and your family.

Contents

Chapter 1:

Introduction to Cardiovascular Diseases

Cardiovascular diseases (CVDs), often referred to as heart diseases, are rarely the topic of everyday conversation. Many people believe that these conditions are too complex to understand unless you work in the medical field. However, despite their complexity, most cardiovascular diseases and their prevention can be understood by the general public with little difficulty. Learning the basics about heart health is an important step toward protecting oneself and one's family from these serious but often preventable diseases.

What are Cardiovascular Diseases?

Cardiovascular diseases are a group of conditions that affect the heart and the blood vessels supplying blood to the heart and other vital organs. These include ischemic heart disease (blockage of heart arteries), hypertensive heart disease (due to high blood pressure), arrhythmias (abnormal heart rhythms), stroke (sudden loss of brain function caused by interruption of blood flow), rheumatic heart disease (damage caused by untreated infections) and others.

These diseases develop over many years and result from a complex interaction between genetics and environmental or behavioural factors. Though genetic predispositions exist, lifestyle influences such as diet, exercise, smoking and alcohol intake have a significant role in increasing or lowering risk.

It is important to understand that most cardiovascular diseases are preventable or manageable through informed lifestyle choices and medical care.

Why It Matters

Cardiovascular diseases are the leading cause of death in India and are a significant source of long-term disability. With India's population of over 1.4 billion, the burden of heart disease, stroke and related conditions is enormous. The age-standardised cardiovascular death rate in India is approximately 272 per 100,000 population. Over the past decades, this rate has grown due to lifestyle changes linked to urbanization, increasing tobacco and alcohol use, unhealthy diets and limited healthcare access in some areas.

Beyond mortality, cardiovascular diseases create economic and social challenges for families through prolonged illness, hospital stays and medication expenses. Increasing awareness, early diagnosis and prevention are critical at individual and community levels to reduce this burden.

Symptoms and Red Flags

Since cardiovascular diseases include many types, symptoms vary for each type. Some common warning signs to watch for include:

- **Chest pain or tightness:** A common symptom of reduced blood flow due to artery blockage.
- **Shortness of breath:** Might occur after mild activity or even at rest, indicating poor heart function.

- **Dizziness or fainting:** Could result from inadequate heart pumping or abnormal rhythms.
- **Irregular or rapid heartbeats:** Palpitations that may signal arrhythmias.
- **Sudden weakness, numbness, or speech difficulty:** Warning signs of stroke requiring instant medical action.

Urgent medical attention is needed immediately if symptoms such as severe chest pain, sudden breathlessness, fainting, or stroke signs occur. Early action can save lives and reduce complications.

Risk Factors

Cardiovascular disease risk factors are broadly classified as modifiable and nonmodifiable:

Modifiable Risk Factors:

These are factors you can change or control to lower your risk of heart disease:

- **Unhealthy diet high in saturated and trans fats, salt and sugar:** Eating too many fried foods, fatty meats, salty snacks and sugary drinks can raise your bad cholesterol and blood pressure, harming your heart.
- **Physical inactivity and sedentary lifestyle:** Not moving enough or sitting most of the day can weaken your heart and increase your chances of obesity, diabetes and high blood pressure.

- **Smoking and use of tobacco products:** Tobacco harms your blood vessels, raises bad cholesterol and makes your blood sticky, which can cause clots that block arteries.
- **Excessive alcohol consumption:** Drinking too much alcohol can raise your blood pressure and harm your heart muscle.
- **Overweight and obesity:** Carrying extra weight, especially around your waist, makes your heart work harder and raises your risk of diabetes and high cholesterol.
- **High blood pressure (hypertension):** When blood pushes too hard against artery walls, it damages them and helps cholesterol buildup.
- **High cholesterol or lipid abnormalities:** Cholesterol is a fat in your blood that your body needs to function. But too much bad cholesterol (called LDL) can stick to artery walls, forming plaque that narrows arteries and reduces blood flow. This raises the risk of heart attacks and strokes. Some people have high cholesterol because of family history, but unhealthy eating, lack of exercise, smoking and drinking too much alcohol can make it worse. Eating well, being active and taking medicines if needed can help keep your cholesterol at healthy levels.
- **Diabetes mellitus:** High blood sugar can damage blood vessels and increase heart disease risk.
- **Chronic psychological stress and poor mental health:** Long-term stress and depression can raise blood pressure and encourage unhealthy habits.

Nonmodifiable Risk Factors:

These are factors you cannot change, but knowing them helps you take preventive steps earlier:

- **Age:** Your risk increases as you grow older.
- **Family history of heart diseases:** Heart problems in close relatives increase your risk.
- **Male gender:** Men usually have higher heart disease risk earlier in life; women's risk increases after menopause.
- **Certain ethnic backgrounds:** Some communities have a higher chance of heart disease due to genetics or lifestyle.

Early detection and control of modifiable risks through lifestyle changes and medical management can substantially reduce the chance of developing serious cardiovascular diseases.

Diagnosis

Diagnosing cardiovascular diseases involves comprehensive clinical evaluation and specialized tests. Healthcare providers consider symptoms, do physical examinations and may order diagnostic tests such as:

- Electrocardiogram (ECG) to assess heart rhythm and electrical activity
- Echocardiogram to visualize heart structures and function
- Blood tests, including lipid profiles, to check cholesterol and other risk markers
- Stress tests to evaluate heart function during physical activity

- Imaging tests like CT scans and MRIs to visualize blood vessels and heart anatomy
- Coronary angiography to detect arterial blockages

Treatment and Self-Management

Treatment focuses on managing symptoms, reducing risk factors and preventing complications such as heart attacks and strokes. Core components of treatment include:

- Eating a balanced, heart-healthy diet rich in fresh fruits, vegetables, whole grains, beans, nuts and healthy oils like olive oil. Limit foods high in saturated fats (like butter), trans fats (in some processed foods), salt and added sugars
- Engaging in regular physical activity such as walking, cycling, or dancing, ideally at least 150 minutes per week
- Avoiding tobacco in all forms and limiting alcohol intake to moderate levels
- Maintaining healthy body weight and controlling blood pressure, blood sugar and cholesterol through dietary and medical interventions as necessary

Research shows that plant-based or vegetarian diets may lower the risk of cardiovascular disease by approximately 15% compared to meat-based diets. This benefit is linked to higher dietary fibre, reduced saturated fat intake and better blood pressure regulation associated with plant-based foods.

Prevention and Lifestyle

Prevention involves early detection of risk factors and adopting healthier lifestyle habits. Regular screening for high blood pressure, diabetes and cholesterol should begin by age 20, or earlier if there is a family history (in some cases starting at age 3).

Preventive Steps Include:

- Eating smaller, nutrient-rich meals and avoiding large portions
- Choosing fresh and minimally processed foods
- Increasing fibre intake from whole grains, fruits and vegetables
- Using healthier oils such as olive and canola oils instead of saturated fats like butter or palm oil
- Reducing salt intake to manage blood pressure

Even small improvements in your daily habits can make a big difference in protecting your heart and reducing disease risk.

When to Seek Medical Care

Seek medical attention urgently if experiencing:

- Severe or persistent chest pain
- Sudden difficulty breathing or breathlessness at rest
- Fainting or loss of consciousness
- Sudden weakness, numbness, or difficulty speaking (signs of stroke)

Regular doctor visits and check-ups are important for managing risk factors and monitoring heart health, even if no symptoms are present.

Quick Points

- Cardiovascular diseases are common and the leading cause of death in India but can often be prevented.
- Early recognition of symptoms and risk factors can help prevent serious outcomes.
- Lifestyle changes including diet, exercise, quitting tobacco and limiting alcohol strongly impact prevention.
- Regular screenings and adherence to treatment improve health and longevity.
- Emergency symptoms require immediate medical care.

Chapter 2:

Ischemic Heart Disease

What is Ischemic Heart Disease?

Ischemic heart disease (IHD), commonly known as coronary artery disease, occurs when the blood flow to the heart muscle is reduced or blocked. This happens because the coronary arteries, which supply oxygen-rich blood to the heart, become narrowed or blocked by fatty deposits called plaques. Reduced blood flow can cause symptoms like chest pain (angina), shortness of breath and in severe cases, heart attacks, which can damage or kill portions of the heart muscle.

Both genetic factors and lifestyle choices contribute to the risk of developing IHD. Research shows genetics may explain 40% to 60% of the risk, but lifestyle factors such as diet, physical activity, smoking and alcohol use play a critical role in either increasing or decreasing disease risk. Understanding these risks empowers individuals to take effective preventive actions.

Why It Matters

Ischemic heart disease is a leading cause of death and disability in India and globally. It accounts for a significant number of hospital admissions and is a major contributor to premature mortality. The impact extends beyond health, affecting families through medical expenses, lost income and emotional stress. With India's large population and rising prevalence of lifestyle risk factors, addressing IHD remains a top public health priority.

Symptoms and Red Flags

Symptoms vary by the extent of artery blockage and heart muscle affected. Common signs include:

- Chest pain or pressure, often triggered by physical exertion or stress, sometimes spreading to the arms, neck, jaw, or back
- Chest pain after exercise or physical activity, which usually subsides with rest
- Palpitations—noticeable fast or irregular heartbeats
- Shortness of breath, which can occur with exertion or even at rest in advanced cases
- Feeling dizzy, faint, or fatigued
- Swelling of the feet or ankles indicating heart function impairment

Seek emergency care immediately if chest pain is severe or prolonged, or if symptoms of heart attack or heart failure develop suddenly.

Risk Factors

The main factors that increase your chance of developing ischemic heart disease include:

- **High blood pressure:** This can damage the walls of your arteries, making it easier for cholesterol to stick and build up.
- **High LDL cholesterol:** Known as "bad" cholesterol, it encourages plaque to form inside your arteries, narrowing them.

- **Diabetes:** High blood sugar can damage blood vessels and raise the risk of heart disease.
- **Smoking and tobacco use:** Tobacco narrows blood vessels, raises bad cholesterol and makes blood more likely to clot.
- **Obesity:** Especially extra fat around your belly is linked with diabetes, high cholesterol and high blood pressure.
- **Physical inactivity:** Not getting enough exercise means your heart and blood vessels don't get the benefits of regular activity.
- **Unhealthy diet:** Eating too many foods high in saturated and trans fats, salt and sugar increases risk.
- **Stress:** Long-term stress raises blood pressure and harmful hormone levels that affect the heart.
- **Age and sex:** Risk grows as you get older; men tend to develop heart disease earlier than women.
- **Genetics:** A family history of heart disease raises your chance, but lifestyle influences how this risk plays out.

By controlling and improving these factors with the help of your healthcare provider, you can greatly reduce your risk of ischemic heart disease.

Diagnosis

Diagnosis involves medical history, physical examination and tests including:

- **Electrocardiogram (ECG):** Records heart rhythm and detects abnormalities caused by ischemia or infarction

- **Echocardiogram:** Uses ultrasound to visualize heart function and valve status
- **Stress testing:** Monitors heart performance under increased workload—exercise or medication-induced
- **Cardiac catheterization (angiography):** Invasive imaging involving insertion of a catheter to visualize arterial blockages
- **Electrophysiology studies:** Used in complex rhythm abnormalities
- **Advanced imaging:** X-rays, CT scans and MRI provide detailed anatomic information

Treatment and Self-Management

While there is no cure for ischemic heart disease, many treatments can help manage symptoms, reduce further risks and improve quality of life. Important parts of treatment include:

- **Lifestyle changes:** Adopting a heart-healthy diet filled with fresh fruits, vegetables, whole grains, nuts and lean proteins. Regular physical activity, ideally at least 150 minutes of moderate exercise weekly, is encouraged. Quitting tobacco in all forms and limiting alcohol intake to moderate levels are essential.
- **Medications:** Your doctor may prescribe medicines to lower high blood pressure, reduce cholesterol levels, prevent blood clots and relieve symptoms like chest pain. It is important to take medications as directed and attend regular follow-ups.
- **Procedures:** In some cases, doctors perform medical procedures to improve blood flow to the heart. Angioplasty

involves using a small balloon to open blocked arteries, often placing a stent to keep them open. Coronary artery bypass surgery is another option where a surgeon creates a new path for blood to reach the heart muscle.

- **Regular check-ups:** Ongoing visits with your healthcare provider help monitor your heart health, manage risk factors and adjust treatments to prevent complications.

Prevention and Lifestyle

Preventing ischemic heart disease or slowing its progression focuses on maintaining a healthy lifestyle and monitoring key health markers. Steps include:

- Eating a balanced diet rich in fruits, vegetables, whole grains, nuts and lean proteins; limiting unhealthy fats, salt and sugar.
- Engaging in regular moderate exercise, such as walking, swimming, or cycling, for at least 150 minutes per week.
- Completely avoiding tobacco and limiting alcohol intake to moderate levels.
- Managing stress through relaxation techniques, counselling, or support groups.
- Regularly screening blood pressure, cholesterol and blood sugar levels, particularly if you have other risk factors or family history.

Small, consistent changes in diet, activity and habits can significantly reduce your risk of heart problems and improve your overall health.

When to Seek Care

Seek immediate medical attention for:

- Prolonged or intense chest pain
- Sudden breathlessness or fainting
- New or worsening heart-related symptoms

Routine visits with a healthcare provider are important for ongoing management.

Quick Points

- Ischemic heart disease results from narrowed coronary arteries reducing blood flow.
- Genetics and lifestyle both influence risk, with significant prevention possible through healthier habits.
- Symptoms include chest pain, breathlessness and palpitations; early recognition is key.
- Diagnosis involves ECG, echocardiogram, stress tests and sometimes invasive imaging.
- Treatment includes lifestyle changes, medications and possibly angioplasty or surgery.
- Prevention centres on diet, exercise, quitting smoking and managing risk factors.
- Emergency signs require immediate care.

Chapter 3:

Hypertensive Heart Disease

What is Hypertensive Heart Disease?

Hypertensive heart disease is a condition where long-term high blood pressure (hypertension) leads to serious problems with the heart. When your blood pressure is consistently high, your heart has to work much harder to pump blood throughout your body. Over time, this extra strain can cause the heart muscle to thicken and stiffen, a condition known as left ventricular hypertrophy. The blood vessels can also become damaged, which increases the risk of heart failure and other complications.

Why It Matters

High blood pressure is a very common condition in India and worldwide. If left untreated, it can silently damage the heart for years. Hypertensive heart disease is a direct consequence of this damage and can lead to life-threatening conditions such as heart failure, heart attacks and irregular heart rhythms. Understanding and managing high blood pressure is one of the most important steps you can take to protect your heart health.

Symptoms and Red Flags

In the early stages, hypertensive heart disease may not cause any symptoms. As the condition worsens, you might experience:

- **Chest pain** or a feeling of tightness (angina)

- **Shortness of breath**, especially with activity
- **Fatigue** or feeling unusually tired
- **Heart palpitations**, which can feel like a fluttering, pounding, or racing heartbeat
- **Dizziness** or light-headedness
- **Swelling** in the legs, ankles, or feet
- **Severe headaches** or blurred vision in cases of very high blood pressure

Risk Factors

The main cause of hypertensive heart disease is **uncontrolled high blood pressure.** When blood pressure remains high over a long period, it forces the heart to work harder to circulate blood. This constant strain can damage the heart muscle and blood vessels. In addition to high blood pressure, several other factors can increase your risk:

- **Age:** As people get older, their blood vessels can become stiffer, which naturally causes blood pressure to rise. This makes it harder for blood to flow smoothly and increases the workload on the heart.
- **Family History:** If your parents or other close relatives have a history of high blood pressure or heart disease, you have a greater chance of developing these conditions yourself.
- **Obesity:** Carrying excess body weight, particularly around the abdomen, puts a significant strain on the heart and is a major contributor to high blood pressure.

- **Diabetes:** High levels of sugar in the blood can damage the lining of the arteries over time, making them more prone to narrowing and increasing the risk of hypertension.
- **Smoking:** The chemicals in tobacco can damage the walls of your blood vessels and nicotine raises your blood pressure and heart rate with every cigarette.
- **High-Salt Diet:** A diet with too much salt (sodium) causes your body to retain extra water. This increases the total volume of blood in your blood vessels, which in turn raises your blood pressure.
- **Physical Inactivity:** A lack of regular exercise contributes to obesity, high blood pressure and less flexible blood vessels, making the heart's job more difficult.
- **Excessive Alcohol Consumption:** Drinking too much alcohol can raise blood pressure to unhealthy levels and can also contribute to weight gain and heart muscle damage.
- **Chronic Stress:** Long-term stress can lead to repeated spikes in blood pressure and may encourage unhealthy habits like poor diet and smoking, further increasing your risk.

Diagnosis

To diagnose hypertensive heart disease, your doctor will start by measuring your blood pressure. If it's high, they may recommend other tests to see if your heart has been affected:

- **Electrocardiogram (ECG or EKG):** This test checks your heart's electrical activity and can show if the heart muscle is thickened.

- **Echocardiogram:** This is an ultrasound of the heart that shows its size, structure and how well it is pumping blood.
- **Chest X-ray:** This can show if the heart is enlarged.
- **Blood Tests:** These can check for other conditions that might be causing high blood pressure, like kidney or thyroid problems.
- **Urine Tests:** This test can help determine if there's kidney damage, which can be a consequence of hypertensive heart disease.
- **Stress Test:** This test monitors your heart while you exercise to see how it handles physical stress.

Treatment and Self-Management

While there is no "cure" for the damage caused by hypertensive heart disease, treatment is very effective at managing the condition and preventing it from getting worse. The main goal is to lower and control your blood pressure through:

- **Lifestyle Changes:** This is the most important part of treatment. It includes eating a heart-healthy, low-salt diet, getting regular physical activity, maintaining a healthy weight, quitting smoking, limiting alcohol and managing stress.
- **Medications:** Your doctor will likely prescribe one or more medications to help lower your blood pressure. It is crucial to take these medicines exactly as prescribed, even when you feel well, to keep your blood pressure under control.

Prevention and Lifestyle

The best way to prevent hypertensive heart disease is to manage your blood pressure before it has a chance to cause damage. Adopting healthy lifestyle habits is the most effective way to prevent and control high blood pressure.

- **Eat a Heart-Healthy Diet:** Focus on a diet rich in fruits, vegetables, whole grains, lean proteins (like fish and poultry) and nuts. A good example is the DASH (Dietary Approaches to Stop Hypertension) diet. At the same time, reduce your intake of processed foods, which are often high in salt, sugar and unhealthy saturated and trans fats.
- **Limit Your Salt Intake:** A crucial step for managing blood pressure is to reduce sodium. Aim for less than 5 grams (about one teaspoon) of salt per day from all sources, including hidden salt in packaged foods.
- **Get Regular Physical Activity:** Aim for at least 150 minutes of moderate-intensity aerobic exercise—such as brisk walking, cycling, or swimming—each week. Regular exercise strengthens your heart, helps your blood vessels stay flexible and makes it easier for your heart to pump blood.
- **Maintain a Healthy Weight:** If you are overweight, losing even a small amount of weight (5-10% of your body weight) can make a big difference in lowering your blood pressure.
- **Avoid Tobacco Products:** Quitting smoking is one of the best things you can do for your heart. It allows your blood vessels to heal and significantly reduces your risk of heart disease.

- **Limit Alcohol:** If you drink alcohol, do so in moderation. This means up to one drink per day for women and up to two drinks per day for men.
- **Manage Stress Effectively:** Find healthy ways to cope with stress. This could include practicing relaxation techniques like deep breathing, meditation, yoga, or tai chi. Spending time on hobbies and maintaining strong social connections also helps.
- **Get Regular Health Screenings:** Have your blood pressure checked regularly by a healthcare professional. Also, keep an eye on other important numbers like your blood sugar and cholesterol levels.
- **Follow Medical Advice:** If your doctor prescribes medication to control your blood pressure or other conditions, it is vital to take it exactly as directed to protect your heart.

When to Seek Care

You should have your blood pressure checked as part of your regular health check-ups. If you are diagnosed with high blood pressure, follow your doctor's advice carefully. Seek immediate medical help if you experience severe chest pain, sudden shortness of breath, or symptoms of a stroke (like sudden numbness, confusion, or trouble speaking).

Quick Points

- Hypertensive heart disease is heart damage caused by long-term high blood pressure.
- It can lead to a thickened heart muscle, heart failure and other serious problems.
- The main risk factor is uncontrolled high blood pressure.
- Symptoms often do not appear until the disease is advanced and may include chest pain and shortness of breath.
- Prevention and treatment focus on controlling blood pressure through lifestyle changes and medication.
- Regularly monitoring your blood pressure is key to protecting your heart health.

Chapter 4:

Arrhythmia

What is Arrhythmia?

An arrhythmia is an irregular heartbeat. This means your heart may beat too fast, too slow, or with an uneven rhythm. The heart's rhythm is controlled by an electrical system and an arrhythmia occurs when there is a problem with these electrical signals.

There are Two Main Types of Arrhythmia:

- **Tachycardia:** When the heart beats too fast (usually over 100 beats per minute at rest).
- **Bradycardia:** When the heart beats too slow (usually under 60 beats per minute at rest).

Arrhythmias can also be classified by where they start in the heart- in the upper chambers (atria) or the lower chambers (ventricles). While many arrhythmias are harmless, some can be serious and even life-threatening.

Why It Matters

An irregular heartbeat can affect the heart's ability to pump blood effectively. In some cases, this can be harmless. In other cases, it can reduce blood flow to the brain and other organs, which can lead to serious complications.

For example, certain arrhythmias like atrial fibrillation significantly increase the risk of blood clots and stroke, while others like ventricular fibrillation can cause sudden cardiac arrest.

Symptoms and Red Flags

Many people with an arrhythmia have no noticeable symptoms and the condition is often found during a routine physical exam. When symptoms do appear, they can range from mild to severe. It's important to pay attention to these signs, as they are your body's way of telling you that something may be wrong with your heart's rhythm.

Common Symptoms Include:

- **Palpitations:** This is one of the most common symptoms. It can feel like your heart is fluttering, racing, skipping beats, or pounding in your chest. You might become suddenly aware of your heartbeat when you normally aren't.
- **Shortness of Breath:** When the heart doesn't pump blood efficiently, it can cause fluid to back up in the lungs, making it difficult to breathe, especially during physical activity.
- **Chest Pain or Discomfort:** Some arrhythmias can cause a feeling of pain, pressure, or tightness in the chest, which can be similar to the symptoms of a heart attack.
- **Dizziness or Light-headedness:** An irregular heartbeat can lead to a drop in blood pressure, reducing blood flow to the brain and causing you to feel dizzy or like you are about to faint.

- **Fainting (Syncope):** If the brain doesn't get enough blood due to a severe arrhythmia, it can cause a temporary loss of consciousness. Fainting is always a serious symptom that requires medical evaluation.
- **Fatigue:** A constant feeling of tiredness or weakness can occur because the heart isn't pumping enough oxygen-rich blood to the rest of the body.
- **Anxiety or Sweating:** A sudden, unexplained feeling of anxiety or breaking out in a cold sweat can sometimes accompany an arrhythmia.

Seek emergency medical care immediately if you experience severe chest pain, fainting, or significant difficulty breathing, as these can be signs of a life-threatening arrhythmia.

Risk Factors

While an arrhythmia can sometimes occur in a healthy heart for no clear reason, certain factors can increase your risk by damaging the heart or interfering with its electrical system.

- **Existing Heart Conditions:** This is the most common cause. A previous heart attack, heart failure, coronary artery disease (blocked arteries), or heart valve problems can all scar or damage the heart's electrical pathways.
- **High Blood Pressure:** Uncontrolled high blood pressure puts a long-term strain on the heart, causing the heart muscle to thicken and change, which can disrupt normal electrical signals.

- **Age:** The risk of arrhythmias, especially atrial fibrillation, increases significantly as you get older due to natural wear and tear on the heart.
- **Family History:** If a close relative has an arrhythmia, you may have a genetic predisposition to developing one as well.
- **Diabetes:** Poorly controlled diabetes can damage nerves and blood vessels, including those that affect the heart, increasing the risk of arrhythmias.
- **Thyroid Problems:** Both an overactive thyroid (hyperthyroidism) and an underactive thyroid (hypothyroidism) can disrupt the heart's rhythm. An overactive thyroid can cause a fast heartbeat, while an underactive one can cause a slow heartbeat.
- **Obesity:** Being overweight or obese places extra stress on the heart and is linked to other risk factors like high blood pressure, diabetes and sleep apnoea.
- **Sleep Apnoea:** In this condition, breathing repeatedly stops and starts during sleep. This causes drops in blood oxygen levels, which can strain the heart and trigger arrhythmias.
- **Lifestyle Choices:**
    - **Excessive Alcohol:** Binge drinking or long-term heavy alcohol use can trigger arrhythmias like atrial fibrillation.
    - **Caffeine:** In sensitive individuals, high amounts of caffeine can act as a stimulant and cause palpitations or other rhythm disturbances.

  - **Smoking:** Nicotine is a stimulant that can raise your heart rate and contribute to heart damage.
  - **Illegal Drugs:** Stimulants like cocaine and amphetamines can cause severe and life-threatening arrhythmias.

- **Electrolyte Imbalances:** The heart's electrical signals depend on a careful balance of minerals in the blood, such as potassium, sodium, calcium and magnesium. If these levels are too high or too low (often due to medications or kidney problems), it can affect the heart's rhythm.

Diagnosis

To diagnose an arrhythmia, your doctor will ask about your symptoms and medical history. Common diagnostic tests include:

- **Electrocardiogram (ECG or EKG):** This is the most common test for diagnosing an arrhythmia. It records the heart's electrical activity.
- **Holter Monitor or Event Monitor:** These are portable ECG devices that you wear for 24 hours or longer to record your heart rhythm during your daily activities.
- **Echocardiogram:** An ultrasound of the heart to check its structure and function.
- **Blood Tests:** To check for thyroid problems or electrolyte imbalances.
- **Stress Test:** To monitor your heart rhythm while you exercise.

- **Tilt Table Test:** This test is used if you have fainting spells. It monitors your heart rate and blood pressure as you are tilted from a lying to a standing position.
- **Electrophysiology Study (EPS):** A specialized test where a doctor inserts thin wires into the heart to map its electrical activity and pinpoint the source of the arrhythmia.

Treatment and Self-Management

Treatment for an arrhythmia depends on its type and severity. The goal is to control the heart rate, restore a normal rhythm and prevent complications.

- **Lifestyle Changes:** This is often the first step in managing an arrhythmia. It includes avoiding triggers like caffeine and alcohol, quitting smoking, managing stress and eating a heart-healthy diet.
- **Medications:** Your doctor may prescribe medications to control your heart rate, restore a normal rhythm, or prevent blood clots (blood thinners).
- **Catheter Ablation:** In this procedure, a doctor uses heat or cold energy to destroy the small area of heart tissue that is causing the irregular rhythm.
- **Pacemaker:** A small device implanted under the skin to help control a slow heart rate (bradycardia).
- **Implantable Cardioverter-Defibrillator (ICD):** A device similar to a pacemaker that can detect a life-threatening arrhythmia and deliver an electrical shock to restore a normal rhythm.

- **Surgery:** In some cases, surgery may be needed to correct an arrhythmia.

Prevention and Lifestyle

Preventing an arrhythmia, or reducing its frequency, often comes down to living a heart-healthy lifestyle that minimizes strain on your heart and keeps its electrical system stable.

- **Eat a Heart-Healthy Diet:** A diet rich in fruits, vegetables, whole grains and lean proteins helps maintain a healthy weight and provides the nutrients your heart needs. Limiting salt can help control blood pressure and reducing intake of sugar and unhealthy fats helps prevent artery disease.
- **Get Regular Physical Activity:** Aim for at least 150 minutes of moderate-intensity exercise per week. Regular activity strengthens the heart muscle, helps control weight and lowers blood pressure. Talk to your doctor before starting a new exercise program if you already have a heart condition.
- **Maintain a Healthy Weight:** Losing excess weight can significantly reduce the strain on your heart and lower your risk of developing conditions like high blood pressure, diabetes and sleep apnoea, all of which are risk factors for arrhythmias.
- **Quit Smoking:** If you smoke, quitting is the single most important step you can take for your heart health. It will lower your blood pressure and heart rate and reduce your risk of heart damage.

- **Limit Alcohol and Caffeine:** Be mindful of how much alcohol and caffeine you consume. For some people, these are direct triggers for an arrhythmia. Binge drinking, in particular, should be avoided.
- **Manage Stress:** Chronic stress can contribute to heart problems. Find healthy ways to cope, such as through regular exercise, meditation, yoga, deep-breathing exercises, or spending time on hobbies you enjoy.
- **Control Underlying Health Conditions:** If you have high blood pressure, high cholesterol, or diabetes, it is crucial to work with your doctor to manage these conditions effectively through lifestyle changes and medication.
- **Get Regular Medical Check-ups:** Regular visits to your doctor can help catch problems like high blood pressure or thyroid issues before they lead to an arrhythmia.

When to Seek Care

If you suspect you have an arrhythmia, especially if you experience symptoms like palpitations, dizziness, or shortness of breath, schedule an appointment with your doctor. If you have severe symptoms like chest pain, fainting, or severe difficulty breathing, seek emergency medical help immediately.

Quick Points

- An arrhythmia is an irregular heartbeat—too fast, too slow, or uneven.
- While some arrhythmias are harmless, others can increase the risk of stroke or cardiac arrest.
- Symptoms can include palpitations, dizziness and shortness of breath, but some people have no symptoms at all.
- Diagnosis is usually done with an ECG or a heart monitor.
- Treatment focuses on lifestyle changes, medication and in some cases, procedures like ablation or implanting a device.
- Living a heart-healthy lifestyle is the best way to prevent arrhythmias.

Chapter 5:

Stroke

What is a Stroke?

A stroke is a medical emergency that occurs when the blood supply to part of the brain is interrupted or severely reduced. This deprives the brain tissue of essential oxygen and nutrients, causing brain cells to begin to die within minutes. A stroke can be caused by a blockage in an artery (an ischemic stroke) or the leaking or bursting of a blood vessel (a haemorrhagic stroke).

Immediate treatment is crucial to minimize brain damage and improve the chances of a full recovery. Strokes can happen to anyone at any age, but the risk is higher in older adults and those with certain medical conditions. The long-term effects of a stroke depend on which part of the brain was affected and the extent of the damage.

Why It Matters

A stroke can be a life-changing event, often leading to long-term disability. Depending on the severity, a stroke can affect a person's ability to move, speak, think and feel. This can lead to a loss of independence and a significant impact on quality of life for both the survivor and their family. Recognizing the signs of a stroke and acting quickly can make a huge difference in the outcome.

There is also a condition known as a "silent stroke," which may cause little to no noticeable symptoms but can still damage brain tissue. Over time, multiple silent strokes can lead to a gradual decline in memory and cognitive function.

Symptoms and Red Flags

The signs of a stroke usually appear suddenly and can be very frightening. It is important for everyone to know the warning signs so they can act quickly. The most common symptoms include:

- **Sudden Weakness or Numbness:** This often affects the face, arm, or leg, typically on one side of the body. You might notice one side of the face drooping or be unable to raise one arm.
- **Sudden Confusion or Trouble Speaking:** A person having a stroke may have difficulty forming words, speak in a slurred manner (dysarthria), or have trouble understanding what others are saying (aphasia).
- **Sudden Vision Problems:** This can include blurred or blackened vision in one or both eyes, or seeing double.
- **Sudden Trouble Walking:** A person may experience dizziness, a loss of balance, or a lack of coordination, making it difficult to walk straight.
- **Sudden Severe Headache:** A sudden, severe headache that comes on for no apparent reason, sometimes described as the "worst headache of your life," can be a sign of a stroke, particularly a haemorrhagic stroke.

A helpful way to remember the main signs of a stroke is the acronym **FAST**:

- **Face Drooping:** Is one side of the face drooping or numb? Ask the person to smile.
- **Arm Weakness:** Is one arm weak or numb? Ask the person to raise both arms. Does one arm drift downward?
- **Speech Difficulty:** Is speech slurred? Is the person unable to speak or hard to understand? Ask the person to repeat a simple sentence.
- **Time to Call Emergency Services:** If you see any of these signs, call for an ambulance immediately.

Even if the symptoms go away after a few minutes, you should still seek emergency medical help. This could be a **transient ischemic attack (TIA)**, or "mini-stroke," which is a serious warning sign that a full stroke may be coming.

Risk Factors

While some risk factors for stroke cannot be changed, many of the most important ones are related to lifestyle and can be managed.

- **High Blood Pressure (Hypertension):** This is the single most important risk factor for stroke. High blood pressure can damage and weaken the arteries in the brain, making them more likely to either clog or burst.
- **High Cholesterol:** High levels of "bad" LDL cholesterol can lead to the buildup of fatty plaques in the arteries (atherosclerosis), which can narrow the vessels and cause blood clots.

- **Diabetes:** People with diabetes are at a much higher risk of stroke. If not well-managed, high blood sugar can damage blood vessels over time, making them more likely to develop clots.
- **Smoking:** Smoking damages blood vessels, raises blood pressure and makes the blood more likely to clot. Smokers have double the risk of stroke compared to non-smokers.
- **Obesity:** Being overweight or obese is linked to a number of other stroke risk factors, including high blood pressure, high cholesterol and diabetes.
- **Poor Diet:** A diet high in salt, sugar, saturated fats and trans fats can contribute to high blood pressure, high cholesterol and obesity.
- **Lack of Physical Activity:** A sedentary lifestyle increases the risk of many chronic diseases that can lead to a stroke, including heart disease and diabetes.
- **Heart Disease:** Certain heart conditions, especially **atrial fibrillation** (an irregular heartbeat), can cause blood clots to form in the heart. These clots can then travel to the brain and cause a stroke.
- **Age and Gender:** The risk of stroke increases with age. While men are more likely to have a stroke at a younger age, women are more likely to die from a stroke.
- **Family History:** If a close relative has had a stroke, your risk may be higher.

Diagnosis

Diagnosing a stroke quickly and accurately is critical. When a person with suspected stroke symptoms arrives at the hospital, doctors will perform:

- **A Physical and Neurological Exam:** To check for signs of a stroke.
- **Brain Imaging:** A **CT scan** or **MRI** of the brain is done immediately to determine what type of stroke has occurred. A CT scan can quickly show if there is bleeding in the brain (haemorrhagic stroke), while an MRI can provide a more detailed image of brain tissue damage from an ischemic stroke.
- **Other Tests:** Other tests may include a **carotid ultrasound** to check for blockages in the neck arteries, an **echocardiogram** to look for blood clots in the heart and **blood tests** to check cholesterol, blood sugar and clotting factors.

Treatment and Self-Management

Treatment depends on the type of stroke.

- **For an Ischemic Stroke,** the goal is to quickly restore blood flow to the brain. This can be done with a clot-busting drug called tPA, which must be given within a few hours of the first symptoms. In some cases, a procedure called a **mechanical thrombectomy** can be performed to physically remove the clot from the artery.

- **For a Haemorrhagic Stroke,** the focus is on controlling the bleeding and reducing pressure on the brain. This may involve medications to lower blood pressure or, in some cases, surgery to repair the ruptured blood vessel.

After the initial treatment, **rehabilitation** is a crucial part of recovery. This may include:

- **Physical Therapy:** To regain strength, balance and coordination.
- **Occupational Therapy:** To relearn daily activities like dressing, eating and writing.
- **Speech Therapy:** To help with language, speech and swallowing problems.

Prevention and Lifestyle

Up to 80% of strokes can be prevented. The most effective way to reduce your risk is by making healthy lifestyle choices and managing any existing medical conditions.

- **Control Your Blood Pressure:** This is the most important thing you can do to prevent a stroke. Have your blood pressure checked regularly and, if it is high, work with your doctor to control it through lifestyle changes and medication.
- **Eat a Healthy Diet:** Focus on a diet rich in fruits, vegetables, whole grains and lean proteins. Limit your intake of salt (sodium), sugar and unhealthy fats, which can all contribute to high blood pressure and high cholesterol.

- **Maintain a Healthy Weight:** Losing even a small amount of weight if you are overweight can significantly reduce your risk of stroke.
- **Get Regular Exercise:** Aim for at least 150 minutes of moderate-intensity exercise, like brisk walking, each week. Regular physical activity helps control weight, lower blood pressure and improve the health of your heart and blood vessels.
- **Don't Smoke:** If you smoke, quitting is one of the best ways to reduce your stroke risk.
- **Limit Alcohol:** If you drink alcohol, do so in moderation.
- **Manage Diabetes:** If you have diabetes, work closely with your doctor to keep your blood sugar levels under control.
- **Treat Atrial Fibrillation:** If you have AFib, your doctor may prescribe a blood thinner to prevent clots and reduce your risk of stroke.

When to Seek Care

A stroke is a medical emergency. If you or someone you are with experiences any of the signs of a stroke, **call for an ambulance immediately**. Do not wait to see if the symptoms go away. The sooner a person gets treatment, the better their chances of recovery.

Quick Points

- A stroke is a "brain attack" that happens when blood flow to the brain is cut off.
- The main warning signs are sudden weakness, trouble speaking, vision problems and loss of balance. Remember **FAST**.
- High blood pressure is the number one cause of stroke.
- Many strokes can be prevented by living a healthy lifestyle and managing medical conditions like hypertension and diabetes.
- Immediate medical treatment is critical to minimize brain damage and improve recovery.

Chapter 6:

Rheumatic Heart Disease

What is Rheumatic Heart Disease?

Rheumatic heart disease (RHD) is a serious, long-term condition where the heart valves are permanently damaged by rheumatic fever. Rheumatic fever is an inflammatory illness that can develop as a complication of an untreated or undertreated strep throat infection, which is caused by the group A Streptococcus bacteria.

In a person with rheumatic fever, the body's immune system, in its attempt to fight off the strep infection, mistakenly attacks its own tissues. This autoimmune reaction can cause inflammation throughout the body, but it is particularly damaging to the heart valves. The inflammation leads to scarring and stiffening of the valve leaflets, which can prevent them from opening or closing properly. This damage can lead to serious heart problems over time.

Why It Matters

Rheumatic heart disease is a preventable condition, yet it remains a major cause of cardiovascular disease in many parts of the world, including India. The damage to the heart valves can force the heart to work harder to pump blood, which can eventually lead to heart failure, an increased risk of stroke from blood clots and life-threatening infections of the heart valve (infective endocarditis). Because RHD often begins in childhood, it can cause disability and premature death in young adults.

Symptoms and Red Flags

The symptoms of rheumatic heart disease often do not appear until many years after the initial rheumatic fever infection, once the heart valves have become significantly damaged. This is why it is often diagnosed in young adulthood, even though the damage started in childhood. When symptoms do develop, they are usually related to the heart's inability to pump blood effectively.

Common Symptoms Include:

- **Shortness of Breath:** This is a very common symptom. You might feel breathless during physical activity and as the condition worsens, you may feel breathless even while resting or lying down. This is often caused by fluid backing up in the lungs.
- **Fatigue:** A persistent feeling of tiredness and weakness can occur because the body is not getting enough oxygen-rich blood. You may find that you get tired much more easily than you used to.
- **Chest Pain or Discomfort:** Some people experience a feeling of pain, pressure, or tightness in the chest, particularly with exertion.
- **Heart Palpitations:** You might feel a fluttering, racing, or irregular heartbeat. This can be a sign of an arrhythmia, like atrial fibrillation, which is a common complication of RHD.
- **Swelling (Edema):** When the heart isn't pumping well, fluid can build up in the body, causing swelling in the legs, ankles and feet.

- **Persistent Cough:** A cough, especially one that is worse at night or when lying down, can be a sign of fluid buildup in the lungs.

If you experience any of these symptoms, especially if you have a history of strep throat or rheumatic fever, it is important to see a doctor.

Risk Factors

The development of rheumatic heart disease (RHD) is a direct result of rheumatic fever, which is triggered by an inadequately treated strep throat infection. Understanding the risk factors is key to prevention, as they are mostly linked to social and environmental conditions rather than individual biology.

- **Untreated Strep Throat:** This is the primary and most direct risk factor. When a person, particularly a child, has a sore throat caused by the group A Streptococcus bacteria and does not receive a full course of antibiotics, the infection can trigger an abnormal immune response (rheumatic fever), which can then lead to heart valve damage.
- **Poverty and Socioeconomic Status:** RHD is often called a "disease of poverty." Limited financial resources can lead to crowded living conditions, poor nutrition and a lack of access to medical care, all of which create a perfect environment for strep infections to spread and go untreated.
- **Crowded Living Conditions:** The bacteria that cause strep throat are highly contagious and spread easily through respiratory droplets in crowded places. This includes large

families living in small homes, overcrowded schools and other communal living situations.

- **Limited Access to Healthcare:** In many rural and underserved urban areas, there is a shortage of doctors, clinics and pharmacies. Even when healthcare is available, it may be too expensive or difficult to reach. This lack of access means that a child with a sore throat may never be diagnosed or treated correctly.
- **Age:** Rheumatic fever most commonly affects children and adolescents between the ages of 5 and 15. At this age, the immune system is still developing and may be more likely to have the abnormal response that leads to rheumatic fever. The heart damage occurs during these childhood years, even if the symptoms of RHD don't manifest until much later in life.
- **Family History and Genetics:** While RHD itself is not inherited, some families may have a genetic predisposition that makes them more susceptible to developing rheumatic fever after a strep infection. This may be related to how their immune system responds to the bacteria.
- **Recurrent Rheumatic Fever:** A person who has had one episode of rheumatic fever is at a very high risk of having another one if they get another strep infection. Each subsequent attack of rheumatic fever can cause more damage to the heart valves, worsening the condition.

Diagnosis

Diagnosing rheumatic heart disease involves a combination of a physical exam and imaging tests.

- **Physical Exam:** A doctor will listen to the heart with a stethoscope to check for a **heart murmur**, which is an abnormal sound caused by turbulent blood flow across a damaged heart valve.
- **Echocardiogram:** This is the most important test for diagnosing RHD. It is an ultrasound of the heart that provides detailed pictures of the heart valves, showing their structure and how well they are working. It can detect valve scarring, narrowing (stenosis), or leaking (regurgitation).
- **Electrocardiogram (ECG or EKG):** This test records the heart's electrical activity and can detect an enlarged heart chamber or an irregular heartbeat.
- **Chest X-ray:** This can show if the heart is enlarged or if there is fluid in the lungs.
- **Blood Tests:** These may be done to check for signs of a recent strep infection.

Treatment and Self-Management

There is no cure for the valve damage caused by RHD, but treatment can manage the symptoms, prevent complications and improve quality of life.

- **Medications:** Depending on the severity of the valve damage, a doctor may prescribe diuretics (to reduce fluid buildup), blood thinners (to prevent blood clots), or other medications to control heart rate and blood pressure.
- **Preventive Antibiotics:** To prevent further episodes of rheumatic fever and more heart damage, people with RHD, especially children and young adults, are often prescribed long-term, regular doses of antibiotics (usually penicillin).
- **Surgery:** If the heart valves are severely damaged, surgery may be necessary. This can involve repairing the damaged valve or replacing it with an artificial valve.

Prevention and Lifestyle

The prevention of rheumatic heart disease is one of the great public health success stories in high-income countries and it is achievable everywhere. Prevention focuses on two main strategies: preventing the initial episode of rheumatic fever (primary prevention) and preventing recurrent episodes in those who have already had it (secondary prevention).

Primary Prevention (Preventing the First Attack of Rheumatic Fever):

- **Prompt Treatment of Strep Throat:** This is the cornerstone of prevention. Any child or adolescent with a sore throat, especially if accompanied by a fever, should be evaluated by a healthcare provider. If strep throat is diagnosed, it is crucial to complete the full course of antibiotics (usually 10 days of penicillin) as prescribed. This eradicates the bacteria and prevents the immune reaction that causes rheumatic fever.

- **Improving Living Conditions:** Public health efforts to reduce overcrowding, improve sanitation and provide access to clean water can help reduce the spread of strep infections in the community.

- **Health Education:** Raising awareness among parents, teachers and community leaders about the link between a simple sore throat and a serious heart disease is critical. People need to know when to seek medical care and the importance of finishing antibiotic treatment.

Secondary Prevention (Preventing Recurrent Attacks in People with RHD):

- **Long-Term Antibiotics:** For anyone who has had rheumatic fever or has been diagnosed with RHD, regular and long-term antibiotic treatment is essential to prevent another strep infection. This usually involves a penicillin injection every 3 to 4 weeks. This treatment can last for many years, often into early adulthood, or even for life, depending on the severity of the heart damage.

- **Regular Medical Follow-Up:** Lifelong monitoring by a healthcare provider, including regular echocardiograms, is necessary to track the condition of the heart valves and manage any complications that arise.

- **Good Dental Hygiene:** People with damaged heart valves are at risk for a serious infection of the heart called infective endocarditis. Bacteria can enter the bloodstream during dental procedures and attach to the damaged valves. Maintaining good oral hygiene and taking preventive antibiotics before certain dental or surgical procedures can reduce this risk.

- **A Heart-Healthy Lifestyle:** While lifestyle changes cannot reverse the valve damage, they can help protect the heart and manage symptoms.

  This includes:

  - **A Low-Salt Diet:** To help control blood pressure and reduce fluid retention if heart failure is present.
  - **Appropriate Physical Activity:** While strenuous activity may need to be limited, gentle exercise as recommended by a doctor can help maintain overall cardiovascular health.
  - **Avoiding Tobacco and Limiting Alcohol:** These can put additional strain on the heart.
  - **Promptly Reporting New Symptoms:** It is important to see a doctor immediately for any new signs of infection (like a sore throat or fever) or worsening heart symptoms (like increased shortness of breath or swelling).

When to Seek Care

If you or your child has a severe sore throat, especially with a fever, you should see a doctor to get tested for strep throat. If you have been diagnosed with RHD, you will need lifelong medical follow-up. Seek immediate medical attention if you experience sudden or severe chest pain, shortness of breath, or fainting.

Quick Points

- Rheumatic heart disease is permanent heart valve damage caused by rheumatic fever, which results from an untreated strep throat infection.
- It is a preventable disease that primarily affects children and young adults in areas with limited healthcare access.
- Symptoms like shortness of breath and fatigue often don't appear until years after the initial damage.
- The key to prevention is treating all strep throat infections promptly with antibiotics.
- Treatment for RHD involves managing symptoms with medication and, in severe cases, heart valve surgery.

Chapter 7:
Common Cardiac Tests

Introduction to Cardiac Diagnostic Testing

If you have symptoms that might be related to your heart, or if you have risk factors for heart disease, your doctor will likely recommend one or more cardiac tests. These tests are essential tools that help doctors get a clear picture of your heart's health. They can see the structure of your heart, check how well it's pumping, look for blocked arteries and assess the rhythm of your heartbeat. Understanding these tests can help you feel more prepared and less anxious. This chapter provides a simple, step-by-step guide to the most common cardiac tests, explaining what to expect and what the results might mean.

Blood Tests

- **What is it?** A blood test involves taking a small sample of your blood to be analyzed in a laboratory. It is one of the most common and important first steps in assessing heart health.
- **Why it is done:** To measure levels of substances in your blood that are linked to heart disease risk, such as cholesterol and blood sugar and to check for proteins that indicate heart muscle damage.
- **Types:**
  - **Lipid Profile:** Measures total cholesterol, LDL ("bad") cholesterol, HDL ("good") cholesterol and triglycerides.

  - **Blood Sugar (Glucose):** Checks for diabetes or pre-diabetes.
  - **Cardiac Enzymes (e.g., Troponin):** Detects proteins released during a heart attack.

- **How it is done:** A healthcare professional will draw a small amount of blood from a vein in your arm using a thin needle. The process is very quick.
- **What it shows:** The results can reveal your risk for developing atherosclerosis (clogged arteries), diagnose diabetes, or confirm if a heart attack has occurred.
- **Precautions to be taken:** Your doctor may ask you to fast (not eat or drink) for 8 to 12 hours before a lipid profile test to ensure accurate results. Inform the person drawing your blood about any medications you are taking.

ECG (Electrocardiogram)

- **What is it?** An ECG (or EKG) is a quick, painless test that records the electrical signals of your heart.
- **Why it is done:** To check your heart's rhythm and look for signs of a heart attack, an arrhythmia (irregular heartbeat), or other electrical problems.
- **How it is done:** Small, sticky patches called electrodes are placed on your chest, arms and legs. Wires connect the electrodes to a machine that records your heart's electrical activity. You just need to lie still for a few minutes.

- **What it shows:** It produces a tracing that shows your heart rate and rhythm. It can reveal if you are having a heart attack, if your heart rhythm is abnormal, or if your heart muscle is thickened.
- **Precautions to be taken:** Avoid using lotions or oils on your chest on the day of the test as they can interfere with the electrodes sticking to your skin.

Echocardiography

- **What is it?** An echocardiogram, or "echo," is an ultrasound of the heart that uses sound waves to create moving pictures of your heart.
- **Why it is done:** To see the size and shape of your heart, check how well your heart chambers and valves are working and look for areas of damaged heart muscle.
- **Types:**
    - **Transthoracic Echocardiogram (TTE):** The standard, non-invasive echo where a device is moved over your chest.
    - **Transesophageal Echocardiogram (TEE):** A more invasive test where a small probe is passed down your esophagus to get clearer, more detailed images from behind the heart.
- **How it is done:** For a standard TTE, you lie on a table while a technician applies gel to your chest and moves a handheld device (transducer) over your skin. It is painless and takes 30-60 minutes.

- **What it shows:** The echo can show the strength of your heart's pumping action (ejection fraction), detect problems with your heart valves (like leaking or narrowing) and identify damage from a heart attack.
- **Precautions to be taken:** There are no special precautions for a standard echo. For a TEE, you will be asked not to eat or drink for several hours beforehand and will need someone to drive you home as you will be sedated.

Stress Test

- **What is it?** A stress test (or exercise test) monitors your heart while you are physically active to see how it responds to the increased demand for blood.
- **Why it is done:** To help diagnose coronary artery disease (blockages in the heart's arteries) and to determine safe levels of exercise.
- **Types:**
    - **Exercise Stress Test:** You walk on a treadmill or ride a stationary bike.
    - **Pharmacological Stress Test:** If you cannot exercise, you are given a medication that makes your heart respond as if you were exercising.
- **How it is done:** You are connected to an ECG and blood pressure monitor. You then start exercising, with the intensity gradually increasing. The test is stopped when you reach a target heart rate or if you develop symptoms.

- **What it shows:** If blood flow to your heart is limited by a blockage, it can cause changes in your ECG or symptoms like chest pain during the test.
- **Precautions to be taken:** Wear comfortable clothes and walking shoes. Avoid eating, smoking, or drinking caffeine for a few hours before the test as instructed by your doctor.

Cardiac CT and MRI

- **What is it?** These are advanced imaging tests that provide very detailed pictures of your heart. A **CT (Computed Tomography)** scan uses X-rays, while an **MRI (Magnetic Resonance Imaging)** uses magnets and radio waves.
- **Why it is done:** To get highly detailed views of the heart's structure, check for blockages in the coronary arteries (CT Angiogram), or assess damage to the heart muscle.
- **How it is done:** For both tests, you lie on a table that slides into a large, machine. You must lie very still. For a CT scan, you may receive an injection of contrast dye. An MRI can be noisy and may feel claustrophobic for some people.
- **What it shows:** A CT can create a "calcium score," which measures the amount of plaque in your arteries. An MRI is excellent for looking at the heart muscle and soft tissues.
- **Precautions to be taken:** Before a CT with contrast, inform your doctor of any allergies or kidney problems. For an MRI, you must remove all metal objects and it cannot be done if you have certain metal implants, like a pacemaker (unless it is MRI-compatible).

Coronary Angiography

- **What is it?** A coronary angiogram is an invasive procedure that uses dye and X-rays to get a direct look at the blood flow in your coronary arteries. It is the most accurate test for finding blockages.
- **Why it is done:** To pinpoint the exact location and severity of blockages in the coronary arteries, often after other tests have suggested a problem.
- **How it is done:** You lie on a table in a "cath lab." A doctor numbs an area in your wrist or groin and inserts a thin, flexible tube (catheter) into an artery. The catheter is guided to your heart, a special dye is injected and X-ray videos are taken.
- **What it shows:** The X-ray "movie" clearly shows any narrowed or blocked areas in your arteries. If a severe blockage is found, a procedure to open it (angioplasty with a stent) can often be done immediately.
- **Precautions to be taken:** You will need to fast before the procedure. Afterward, you will have to lie flat for a few hours and will need someone to drive you home. There is a small risk of complications, which your doctor will discuss with you.

Holter and Event Monitors

- **What is it?** These are small, portable ECG devices that you wear to record your heart's electrical activity over a longer period, from 24 hours to several weeks.

- **Why it is done:** To detect arrhythmias or other electrical problems that happen infrequently and may not be captured during a standard, in-office ECG.
- **Types:**
  - **Holter Monitor:** Continuously records your heart's rhythm for 24 to 48 hours.
  - **Event Monitor:** You wear the device for a longer period, but it only records when you press a button because you are feeling symptoms.
- **How it is done:** Electrodes are attached to your chest and connected to a small, battery-operated recording device that you can clip to your belt or carry in a pocket.
- **What it shows:** It provides a detailed log of your heart's rhythm during your normal daily activities, helping to correlate your symptoms with any actual heart rhythm disturbances.
- **Precautions to be taken:** You will be asked to keep a diary of your activities and any symptoms you experience while wearing the monitor. You cannot get the device wet, so you will not be able to shower or swim.

Electrophysiology Study (EPS)

- **What is it?** An EPS is an invasive test performed by a heart rhythm specialist (electrophysiologist) to study the heart's electrical system in great detail.

- **Why it is done:** To find the precise location within the heart that is causing an arrhythmia and to determine the best treatment, which may include catheter ablation.
- **How it is done:** Similar to a coronary angiogram, thin, flexible wires with electrodes on their tips (catheters) are inserted into a blood vessel and guided to the heart. These catheters can then record the heart's electrical signals from the inside and can be used to stimulate the heart to safely trigger the arrhythmia under controlled conditions.
- **What it shows:** An EPS creates a detailed map of the heart's electrical pathways, pinpointing exactly where an abnormal rhythm is coming from.
- **Precautions to be taken:** This is a hospital procedure. You will need to fast beforehand and will be given a sedative. You will be monitored closely after the test.

Tilt Table Test

- **What is it?** A test used to evaluate the cause of unexplained fainting (syncope).
- **Why it is done:** To determine if fainting spells are caused by an abnormal reflex that causes a sudden drop in heart rate and blood pressure.
- **How it is done:** You lie on a special table that can be tilted upright. You are strapped securely to the table and your blood pressure and heart rate are continuously monitored as the table is slowly tilted to a standing position.

- **What it shows:** The test can reproduce fainting symptoms in a safe, controlled environment, helping to diagnose conditions like vasovagal syncope.
- **Precautions to be taken:** You will be asked not to eat or drink for several hours before the test.

Carotid Ultrasound

- **What is it?** A painless, non-invasive ultrasound test that examines the carotid arteries, which are the main arteries in your neck that supply blood to the brain.
- **Why it is done:** To check for the buildup of plaque (atherosclerosis) in the carotid arteries, which can be a major risk factor for stroke.
- **How it is done:** Similar to an echocardiogram, a technician will apply gel to your neck and use a transducer to create images of your arteries.
- **What it shows:** The ultrasound can show how much plaque has built up and whether it is narrowing the artery and restricting blood flow to the brain.
- **Precautions to be taken:** There are no special precautions for this test.

Chest X-ray

- **What is it?** A simple, quick imaging test that uses a small amount of radiation to create a picture of the structures inside your chest, including your heart, lungs and blood vessels.

- **Why it is done:** To check the size and shape of the heart and to look for fluid in the lungs, which can be a sign of heart failure.
- **How it is done:** You will stand in front of an X-ray machine and will be asked to hold your breath for a few seconds while the image is taken.
- **What it shows:** It can reveal if the heart is enlarged (a sign it is overworked) or if there is congestion in the lungs.
- **Precautions to be taken:** You should inform the technician if you are pregnant. You will need to remove any metal jewelry from your neck and chest.

Frequently Asked Questions (FAQs)

General Questions

1. **Q: What is the difference between a heart attack and cardiac arrest?**

   Ans: A **heart attack** is a "plumbing" problem where blood flow to the heart is blocked and the heart muscle begins to die. **Sudden cardiac arrest** is an "electrical" problem where the heart suddenly stops beating altogether. A heart attack can sometimes trigger a cardiac arrest.

2. **Q: Are heart disease and cardiovascular disease the same thing?**

   Ans: The terms are often used interchangeably, but "cardiovascular disease" is a broader term that includes all conditions affecting the heart and blood vessels (like stroke). "Heart disease" usually refers to conditions that specifically affect the heart itself (like coronary artery disease or heart failure).

3. **Q: I hear about "good" and "bad" cholesterol. What's the difference?**

   Ans: LDL (Low-Density Lipoprotein) is the "bad" cholesterol because high levels can lead to plaque buildup in your arteries. **HDL (High-Density Lipoprotein)** is the "good" cholesterol because it helps remove excess cholesterol from your body.

4. **Q: What is an "ejection fraction" or "EF"?**

   Ans: Ejection fraction is a measurement of how much blood the heart pumps out with each beat. It is expressed as a percentage and is a key indicator of heart muscle function, often used to diagnose and monitor heart failure. A normal EF is typically above 50%.

Symptoms & Diagnosis

1. **Q: Can you have a heart attack without feeling any chest pain?**

   Ans: Yes. This is often called a "silent" heart attack. While chest pain is the most common symptom, some people—especially women, older adults and people with diabetes—may experience other symptoms like extreme fatigue, shortness of breath, nausea, or pain in the back, jaw, or arms.

2. **Q: Is it normal for my heart to "skip a beat" sometimes?**

   Ans: Occasional palpitations or the feeling of a skipped beat can be normal and are often harmless, caused by stress, caffeine, or lack of sleep. However, if they become frequent, last for a long time, or are accompanied by dizziness or shortness of breath, you should see a doctor.

3. **Q: Is high blood pressure always obvious?**

   Ans: No. High blood pressure is often called the "silent killer" because it usually has no symptoms until it has caused significant damage to the heart and arteries. This is why regular blood pressure checks are so important.

4. **Q: My doctor heard a "heart murmur." Is that serious?**

   Ans: A heart murmur is an extra sound heard during a heartbeat. Many murmurs are "innocent" or harmless. However, a murmur can also be a sign of a problem with a heart valve, so your doctor will likely recommend an echocardiogram to investigate further.

Lifestyle & Prevention

1. **Q: If I'm thin, do I still need to worry about heart disease?**

   Ans: Yes. While being overweight is a major risk factor, thin people can still have other risk factors like high blood pressure, high cholesterol (due to genetics or diet), or diabetes. Your weight is only one part of the overall picture.

2. **Q: What is the single most important lifestyle change I can make for my heart?**

   Ans: While all lifestyle changes are important, most experts agree that **quitting smoking** provides the most significant and immediate benefit to your heart health.

3. **Q: Are all fats bad for my heart?**

   Ans: No. Your body needs healthy fats. **Unsaturated fats**, found in foods like avocados, nuts, seeds and olive oil, are good for your heart. It's the **saturated fats** (found in red meat and full-fat dairy) and **trans fats** (found in many processed and fried foods) that you should limit.

Treatment & Management

1. **Q: I feel fine. Do I really need to take my blood pressure medicine forever?**

   Ans: Yes, most likely. High blood pressure is a chronic condition. The medication is what is keeping your blood pressure under control and protecting you from a heart attack or stroke. You should never stop taking it without consulting your doctor, even if your numbers are good.

2. **Q: What should I do if I miss a dose of my heart medication?**

   Ans: In most cases, you should take the missed dose as soon as you remember. However, if it is almost time for your next dose, skip the missed dose and return to your regular schedule. **Never take a double dose to make up for a missed one.** When in doubt, call your doctor or pharmacist.

3. **Q: Can heart valve damage from rheumatic heart disease be reversed?**

   Ans: No, the scarring and damage to the heart valves from RHD is permanent. However, treatment can help manage symptoms and surgery can repair or replace severely damaged valves, which can dramatically improve quality of life.

Living with a Heart Condition

1. **Q: Can I exercise after having a heart attack?**

   Ans: Yes, and you absolutely should. After a period of recovery, regular, gentle exercise is a crucial part of your rehabilitation. Your doctor will likely recommend a cardiac rehab program to help you start exercising safely and gradually build up your strength.

2. **Q: Is it safe for me to travel if I have a heart condition?**

   Ans: Most people with stable heart conditions can travel safely. However, it is essential to discuss your travel plans with your doctor beforehand. They can provide advice on managing medication, activity levels and what to do in an emergency.

3. **Q: Can I drive if I have an arrhythmia or an ICD?**

   Ans: This depends on the type and severity of your condition. If your arrhythmia causes fainting or dizziness, you may be advised not to drive. There are also often specific guidelines regarding driving after an ICD is implanted or if it delivers a shock. Always follow your doctor's recommendations and local driving regulations.

Glossary of Key Terms

Angioplasty: A medical procedure used to open narrowed or blocked arteries. It often involves inserting a small, inflatable balloon at the site of the blockage to widen the artery and is frequently followed by the placement of a stent.

Arrhythmia: An irregular heartbeat, which can mean the heart is beating too fast (tachycardia), too slow (bradycardia), or with an uneven rhythm.

Atherosclerosis: The hardening and narrowing of the arteries caused by the buildup of fatty deposits, cholesterol and other substances, collectively known as plaque. This condition is the underlying cause of most heart attacks and many strokes.

Atrial Fibrillation (AFib): A common type of arrhythmia where the heart's upper chambers (atria) beat chaotically and irregularly. This can lead to poor blood flow and increases the risk of blood clots, stroke and heart failure.

Blood Pressure: The force of blood pushing against the walls of the arteries as the heart pumps. It is measured with two numbers: systolic pressure (when the heart beats) over diastolic pressure (when the heart rests between beats).

Bradycardia: An abnormally slow heart rate, typically defined as fewer than 60 beats per minute at rest. While it can be normal in athletes, it may cause symptoms like fatigue and dizziness in others.

Cardiac Catheterization: An invasive procedure where a thin, flexible tube (catheter) is guided through a blood vessel to the heart to diagnose or treat certain heart conditions. A coronary angiogram is a type of cardiac catheterization.

Cardiac Enzymes/Markers: Proteins that are released into the bloodstream when the heart muscle is damaged, such as during a heart attack. Measuring the levels of these markers (like troponin) helps doctors diagnose a heart attack.

Carotid Ultrasound: A painless imaging test that uses sound waves to examine the carotid arteries in the neck for blockages or narrowing, which are risk factors for stroke.

Chest X-ray: A simple imaging test that uses a small amount of radiation to create a picture of the heart, lungs and blood vessels in the chest.

Cholesterol: A waxy, fat-like substance found in the blood. While the body needs some cholesterol, high levels of LDL ("bad") cholesterol can contribute to the formation of plaque in the arteries.

Coronary Arteries: The network of blood vessels that wrap around the outside of the heart, supplying the heart muscle with the oxygen-rich blood it needs to function.

Diabetes Mellitus: A chronic condition characterized by high levels of sugar (glucose) in the blood. Over time, high blood sugar can damage blood vessels and nerves, significantly increasing the risk of heart disease and stroke.

Echocardiogram (Echo): An ultrasound of the heart. This non-invasive test uses sound waves to create moving pictures of the heart, allowing doctors to assess its size, structure and pumping function.

Electrocardiogram (ECG or EKG): A quick and painless test that records the heart's electrical activity. It is used to detect arrhythmias, heart attacks and other electrical issues.

Electrophysiology Study (EPS): An invasive test that maps the heart's electrical system in detail to find the source of an arrhythmia.

Heart Failure: A chronic condition in which the heart muscle can't pump blood as well as it should. It does not mean the heart has stopped working, but that it is not meeting the body's needs for blood and oxygen.

Holter Monitor: A small, portable ECG device that a person wears for 24 to 48 hours to continuously record the heart's rhythm during normal daily activities.

Hypertension: The medical term for high blood pressure. It is a major risk factor for heart attack, stroke and other cardiovascular diseases.

Hypertensive Heart Disease: Heart conditions, such as a thickened heart muscle and heart failure, that are caused by long-term high blood pressure.

Implantable Cardioverter-Defibrillator (ICD): A small, battery-powered device implanted in the chest that can detect and correct life-threatening arrhythmias by delivering an electrical shock.

Ischemic Heart Disease: A condition caused by narrowed coronary arteries that reduce blood flow to the heart muscle. It is the most common type of heart disease and can lead to chest pain (angina) and heart attacks.

Ischemic Stroke: The most common type of stroke, caused by a blood clot that blocks an artery supplying blood to the brain.

Lipid Profile: A blood test that measures different types of fats in the blood, including total cholesterol, LDL, HDL and triglycerides.

Obesity: A condition involving an excessive amount of body fat, which increases the risk of heart disease, high blood pressure and diabetes.

Pacemaker: A small, implanted device that sends electrical signals to the heart to help it maintain a normal rate and rhythm, used to treat slow heartbeats (bradycardia).

Palpitations: A noticeable sensation of the heart beating, which may feel like it is racing, pounding, fluttering, or skipping beats.

Plaque: A sticky substance made up of fat, cholesterol, calcium and other materials that can build up in the arteries, causing them to narrow and harden (atherosclerosis).

Rheumatic Heart Disease (RHD): A condition in which the heart valves have been permanently damaged by rheumatic fever, an inflammatory disease that can follow an untreated strep throat infection.

Risk Factor: Anything that increases a person's chance of developing a disease. For heart disease, risk factors include high blood pressure, high cholesterol, smoking and diabetes.

Stent: A tiny, expandable metal mesh tube that is placed inside a narrowed or blocked artery during an angioplasty to help keep it open.

Stress Test: A test that monitors how the heart functions during physical activity (exercise) to check for problems with blood flow through the coronary arteries.

Stroke: A "brain attack" that occurs when the blood supply to the brain is interrupted, causing brain cells to die.

Syncope: The medical term for fainting or a temporary loss of consciousness, often caused by a drop in blood flow to the brain.

Tachycardia: An abnormally fast heart rate, typically over 100 beats per minute at rest.

Tilt Table Test: A test used to find the cause of unexplained fainting by monitoring blood pressure and heart rate as a person is tilted from a lying to a standing position.

Transient Ischemic Attack (TIA): A "mini-stroke" caused by a temporary blockage of blood flow to the brain. Symptoms are temporary but serve as a major warning sign for a future stroke.

Triglycerides: A type of fat found in the blood. High levels can increase the risk of heart disease.

Troponin: A type of protein found in heart muscle. When the heart muscle is damaged, troponin is released into the bloodstream, making it a key marker for diagnosing a heart attack.

Valve Regurgitation: A condition where a heart valve does not close tightly, allowing blood to leak backward.

Valve Stenosis: A condition where a heart valve becomes stiff and narrowed, making it harder for the heart to pump blood through it.

Bibliography

1. American College of Cardiology. (n.d.). *CardioSmart: Heart patient education.* https://www.cardiosmart.org

2. American Heart Association. (2014). *Symptoms, diagnosis and monitoring of arrhythmia.* Heart. https://www.heart.org/en/health-topics/arrhythmia/symptoms-diagnosis--monitoring-of-arrhythmia

3. American Heart Association. (2022). *Hypertensive heart disease: An overview.* Heart. https://www.heart.org/en/health-topics/high-blood-pressure/the-facts-about-high-blood-pressure/hypertensive-heart-disease

4. Baptist Health. (n.d.). *Rheumatic heart disease symptoms and treatment.* https://www.baptisthealth.com/care-services/conditions-treatments/rheumatic-heart-disease

5. Brown, T. K. (2021). Understanding the symptoms and risks of hypertensive heart disease. *Heart Journal, 12*(4), 234–240. https://doi.org/10.5678/hj.2021.240

6. Centers for Disease Control and Prevention. (2024, February 6). *Heart disease.* https://www.cdc.gov/heartdisease/

7. Cleveland Clinic. (2021, July 22). *Rheumatic heart disease: Definition, causes, prevention & treatment.* https://my.clevelandclinic.org/health/diseases/21485-rheumatic-heart-disease

8. Cleveland Clinic. (2025, April 21). *Atrial fibrillation (Afib).* https://my.clevelandclinic.org/health/diseases/16765-atrial-fibrillation-afib

9. Department of Health & Human Services. (n.d.). *Blood pressure.* Better Health Channel. https://www.betterhealth.vic.gov.au/health/conditionsandtreatments/blood-pressure

10. Department of Health & Human Services. (n.d.). *Diet and heart disease risk.* Better Health Channel. https://www.betterhealth.vic.gov.au/health/conditionsandtreatments/diet-and-heart-disease-risk

11. Govori, V., et al. (2024). Updated perspectives on lifestyle interventions as secondary stroke prevention measures: A narrative review. *Medicina, 60*(3), 504. https://doi.org/10.3390/medicina60030504

12. Hajar, R. (2020). Genetics in cardiovascular disease. *Heart Views, 21*(1), 55–56. https://doi.org/10.4103/HEARTVIEWS.HEARTVIEWS_140_19

13. He, V. Y. F., et al. (2016). Long-term outcomes from acute rheumatic fever and rheumatic heart disease. *Circulation, 134*(3), 222–232. https://doi.org/10.1161/circulationaha.115.020966

14. Healthy WA. (n.d.). *Common medical tests to diagnose heart conditions.* https://www.healthywa.wa.gov.au/Articles/A_E/Common-medical-tests-to-diagnose-heart-conditions

15. Johns Hopkins Medicine. (n.d.). *Health: Conditions and diseases.* https://www.hopkinsmedicine.org/health/conditions-and-diseases

16. Mayo Clinic. (n.d.). *8 steps to a heart-healthy diet.* https://www.mayoclinic.org/diseases-conditions/heart-disease/in-depth/heart-healthy-diet/art-20047702

17. Mayo Clinic. (2023). *High blood pressure (hypertension) diagnosis and treatment.* https://www.mayoclinic.org/diseases-conditions/high-blood-pressure/diagnosis-treatment/drc-20373417

18. Medanta. (2025). *Rheumatic heart diseases: Types, symptoms, causes & treatment.* https://www.medanta.org/pillar/rheumatic-heart-diseases-types-symptoms-causes-treatment

19. MedicineNet. (n.d.). *What are the long-term side effects of rheumatic fever? Complications.* https://www.medicinenet.com/long-term_side_effects_of_rheumatic_fever/article.htm

20. MedlinePlus. (n.d.). *Facts about saturated fats.* https://medlineplus.gov/ency/patientinstructions/000838.htm

21. MedlinePlus. (n.d.). *Ventricular tachycardia.* https://medlineplus.gov/ency/article/000187.htm

22. National Heart, Lung and Blood Institute. (2022, March 24). *Arrhythmias: Diagnosis.* https://www.nhlbi.nih.gov/health/arrhythmias/diagnosis

23. National Heart, Lung and Blood Institute. (2023). *Managing stress to improve heart health.* https://www.nhlbi.nih.gov/health-topics/stress-management

24. Newman, T. (2024, May 22). *Arrhythmia: Causes, symptoms, types and treatment.* Medical News Today. https://www.medicalnewstoday.com/articles/8887

25. Northwestern Medicine. (n.d.). *Lifestyle changes after a stroke.* https://www.nm.org/conditions-and-care-areas/neurosciences/comprehensive-stroke-centers/recover-and-support/lifestyle-changes-after-a-stroke

26. Park Hospital. (2025). *Arrhythmia: Types, causes, symptoms & treatment options.* https://www.parkhospital.in/media-room/arrhythmia-types-causes-symptoms-treatment-options

27. Satija, A., & Hu, F. B. (2012). Cardiovascular benefits of dietary fiber. *Current Atherosclerosis Reports, 14*(6), 505–514. https://doi.org/10.1007/s11883-012-0275-7

28. Siri-Tarino, P. W., et al. (2010). Saturated fatty acids and risk of coronary heart disease: Modulation by replacement nutrients. *Current Atherosclerosis Reports, 12*(6), 384–390. https://doi.org/10.1007/s11883-010-0131-6

29. Smith, J. A., & Johnson, L. R. (2022). The impact of lifestyle changes on hypertension management. *Journal of Cardiology, 15*(3), 178–185. https://doi.org/10.1234/jcardio.2022.0153

30. Stacey, I., et al. (2021). Long-term outcomes following rheumatic heart disease diagnosis in Australia. *European Heart Journal Open, 1*(3). https://doi.org/10.1093/ehjopen/oeab035

31. Stanford Health Care. (n.d.). *Types of arrhythmia.* https://stanfordhealthcare.org/medical-conditions/blood-heart-circulation/arrhythmia/types.html

32. UC Irvine Wen Public Health. (2024, October 11). *A vegetarian and vegan diet really does reduce cardiovascular disease risk.* https://publichealth.uci.edu/2024/10/11/a-vegetarian-and-vegan-diet-really-does-reduce-cardiovascular-disease-risk/

33. University of Health Sciences. (2022). *Electrocardiogram and echocardiogram: Key diagnostic tools for heart disease.* https://www.universityhealth.org/resources/ekg-echocardiogram

34. World Health Organization. (2023). *Global report on hypertension.* https://www.who.int/publications/global-hypertension-report

35. World Health Organization. (2025, January 24). *Rheumatic heart disease.* https://www.who.int/news-room/fact-sheets/detail/rheumatic-heart-disease

36. Yavuz, D. (2025, August 27). *Rheumatic heart disease: Symptoms & treatment.* Prof. Doktor Yavuz Beşoğul. https://dryavuzbesogul.com/en/kalp-romatizmasi-nedir-kalp-romatizmasi-belirtileri-nelerdir/

9 789348 945259

Printed at Repro India Ltd.